Mantras for Change & Healing

LEVERAGING NEUROPLASTICY & REPETITION FOR HEALTH AND WELLBEING

Ryan Scott Shannon

Table of Contents

I Am Capable of Change Right Here, Right Now

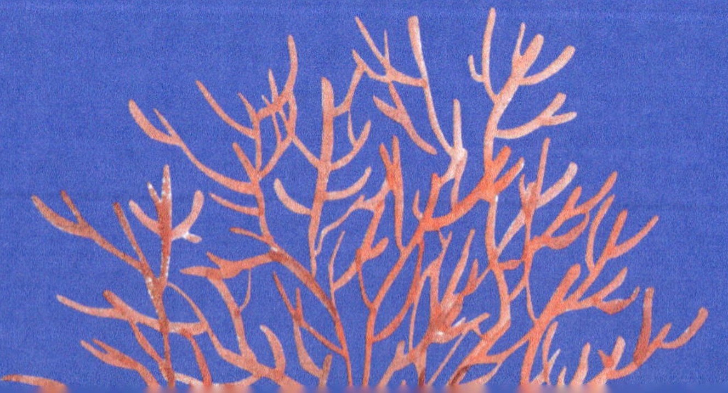

You Are Capable of Change

"A particular train of thought persisted in, be it good or bad, cannot fail to produce its results on the character and circumstances. A man cannot directly choose his circumstances, but he can choose his thoughts, and so indirectly, yet surely, shape his circumstances."
— James Allen, As a Man Thinketh

Do you feel stuck in life?
Do you constantly neglect your resolutions?
Are you looking for ways to defeat harmful or self-defeating behaviors?

That's where mantras come in. Mantras are an important tool when it comes to changing behavior. And while it may seem insignificant, repeating important phrases to yourself can help to hardwire certain positive behaviors you desire. In other words, you are capable of change. With the discovery of plasticity in the brain, there's now scientific backing that thoughts can help to rewire learned behaviors, and can even change the physical structure of the brain.

While there are certain parts of ourselves that can't be changed, such as our genetics and our experiences, neuroplasticity has revealed there's much we can do to train our brains and central nervous system, and therefore our behavior, too. If you feel like you're stuck, and that you can't beat certain bad behaviors, such as overeating or feeling anxious in social settings, just know that there is hope. While mantras may not solve all your problems and aren't a magical cure-all, they can help chip away at neural pathways carved out in your brain to foster new, better habits.

Remember that change is a natural part of being human. Throughout the course of our lives, we may change our beliefs, behaviors, attitudes, and habits. While some changes may be harder than others, with a bit of determination and motivation (and the implementation of tools, such as mantras) you can become a better you. Now, it's time to ditch those bad habits and become a happier, healthier you!

Introduction to Mantras

Are you feeling unmotivated when it comes to your health goals?

Do you feel like your beliefs hold you back from being a better you?

Are you tired of not making meaningful changes that stick?

If so, mantras can help you! There's convincing research that mediation techniques, including the use of mantras, can help reduce stress and possibly help you make more rational, objective decisions. If you'd like to help reprogram your inner beliefs so that they better suit your healing goals, then this is the book for you.

This book is split up into four main sections: 1. Creating change right here, right now 2. Future self-visualizations 3. Radical gratitude and awe, and 4. Entrusting the mysteries and science of the body. These four sections combine to help overhaul your current beliefs surrounding your body and hopefully replace them with the belief that you are strong, capable of change and accepting of your body no matter its condition.

Within each section, you'll receive several mantras as well as a breakdown to help you better digest them. These mantras can be spoken aloud to yourself in a quiet room or can be read and reread in your head.

Not only, you'll also be given mindfulness-infused exercises after receiving each mantra to help the mantra "stick". These exercises are inspired by "Anapana" and "Vipassana" meditation techniques that help you to realize everything is transient, including the negative feelings you may harbor towards yourself and your body.

I hope this book of mantras is insightful, inspiring, and leads to positive changes in your life.

Mantras… Quackery? Or an Effective Strategy to Train the Brain?

Mantras…Quackery? Or an Effective Strategy to Train the Brain?

Wait, how can mantras help you heal? You may be asking yourself this question. While it may seem like quackery, there is some convincing evidence that supports the effectiveness of mantras. Reciting mantras can help reduce symptoms of post-traumatic stress disorder, manage stress, and build resilience (Oman et al, 2022). And meditation, in general, has a range of benefits that you may be aware of, including: decreased blood pressure, even in those with hypertension; increased energy levels; better immune system function (Hyland et al., 2015); and even improved work satisfaction (Hülsheger & Alberts, 2020).

With so much information—and disinformation—out there, it can be hard to decipher fact from fiction when it comes to your health. One day saturated fats are bad for you, the next they're discovered to be an important fatty acid found in human breast milk and a necessary precursor to sex hormones like testosterone, estrogen, and progesterone. One day cholesterol clogs the arteries, the next it's necessary for maintaining cell membranes, acts as a precursor to vitamin D production, and can help repair inflammation-induced damage.

With so much flip-flopping, how can you be sure mantras will be beneficial to you? First, mantras have been safely and effectively used for thousands of years in both Eastern and Western cultures. Next, the scientific literature on mantras, prayer and meditation is robust (more on this in the upcoming section).

I don't mean to add to the confusion by mentioning these health contradictions that are spouted off at us. Rather, I hope to show you that the ultimate power lies in you. You decide what goes into your body. You decide what you value. You decide what's credible. You're the ultimate authority over your life. Whether that means resorting to the analytical mind and combing through PubMed to find studies that support a hypothesis you've built up in your mind, or simply relying on deep-seated intuition, the solutions lie within you.

Let these mantras be a way to help you rediscover your innate healing capabilities and put your mind at ease. I hope these serve as tools to help you return to a state of ease rather than disease.

Sorting Through the Chaos

You may be wondering how reciting some words a few times a day will make a difference in your journey towards better health and becoming a better you. While it may seem very *woo-woo*, mantras can help you access your highest self. The self that helps you navigate the ever-changing health fads and misinformation.

Regular repetition will create new connections in the brain, allowing you to kick your old habits that have been encoded into the subconscious mind. In fact, this idea is supported by a study on mantras and PTSD among war veterans; it was found that a higher frequency of mantra practice was associated with better clinical outcomes, including less severe PTSD symptoms and decreased anger ([Malaktaris et al, 2022](#)). In essence, by utilizing mantras, you'll be upgrading your subconscious mind with new, higher values.

It's thought that in our infancy (ages zero to six) we're nothing but sponges. This is when our programming is installed. Everything from the language we speak, to the way we form romantic relationships (i.e. Attachment Style Theory), to personality is thought to be encoded during this critical life stage. You've probably received some programming throughout your life (especially from childhood) that has influenced your values—and not for the better.

Remember those fast food commercials that would play during your favorite cartoons? Your favorite athletes' faces on sugary cereals? The magazines that tricked you into believing there are shortcuts and miracle pills to help keep you thin? These are just a few examples of the way predatory marketing practices and lax government regulation may have tarnished your subconscious mind and values.

Sadly, many involved in pharmaceuticals (including immoral doctors) have a vested interest in dissuading the masses. Whistleblower Carlat, M.D. reveals in his book, "Unhinged: The Trouble with Psychiatry" that many other psychiatrists push ineffective drugs rather than practice psychotherapy. More sick people on drugs means more money. As of now, the total nominal spending on pharmaceuticals in 2019 was 511.4 billion dollars (Statista, 2019).

Unlike many doctors, I'm not selling you anything. Rather, my goal in writing these mantras and disseminating this information to you is to help you and others make positive changes on a micro level so that we all benefit at a macro level.

In other words, when you make your health and bettering your life a priority, you're playing a key role in making the world a better place. Unlike those pesky commercials for medications that are constantly aired on TV, I make virtually no money from the information I provide (just a few dollars). There's no financial incentive for me to write this book; I'm doing it to help you help yourself.

Now, before we start reciting mantras, I want to go over why mantras can help you. There's no way mantras can have powerful physiological effects on the body, right?

Turns out, they can!

Reciting a few words throughout the day with intention will almost magically help you upgrade the current version of yourself. *Abrakadabra!* This popular, magical phrase stems from Aramaic, meaning "I will create as I speak." Your words, mantras, and prayers are powerful spells that direct your actions (that's why you should always be careful of how you speak of yourself and others).

Now, let's cover the science of mantras.

The Science Behind Mantras, Prayers & Meditations

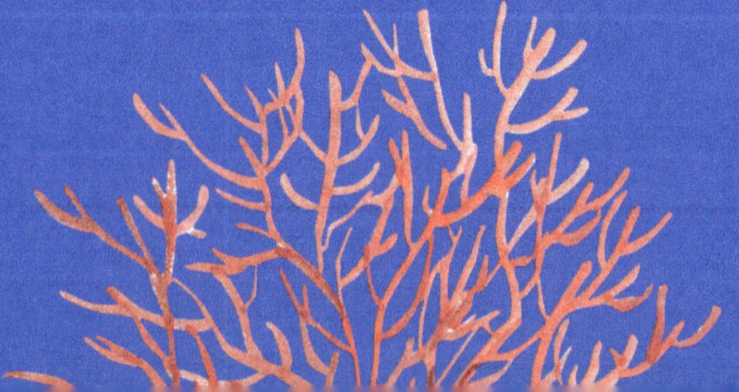

The Science Behind Mantras, Prayers, and Affirmations

To believe something, it's got to make sense. While it may seem crazy to think that meditation and mantras can lead to a better body and health, you'll understand through the following summaries of studies how reduced stress, lowered inflammation, and increased cognition can lead to a better you. The studies prove mantras, meditation and prayers are highly effective in achieving physical changes—it really may be mind over matter after all!

Mantras are similar to prayers in that they're both typically short statements that help you to align with higher values that are usually said throughout the day. I decided to use 'mantra' in the title rather than 'prayer' since 'mantra' doesn't have a religious connotation, however, we can think of them as almost the same. Instead of the "Hail Mary" for Catholics, the "Shema" for Jews, and the "Shahada" for Muslims, mantras can be thought of as universal prayers for those of any—or no—religious affiliation.

- **Significant brain changes were found in 78 studies**. In a meta-analysis, neuroimaging studies involving the brain activity of subjects while meditating (which included mantra meditation) were compared to control groups. This meta-analysis concluded that the "insula, frontopolar cortex and dorsal anterior cingulate" were all activated during meditation (Fox et al, 2016).

- **Curbs cortisol which is associated with chronic inflammation, depression and disease**. Cortisol has entered common parlance in recent years for good reason. While cortisol is an important hormone necessary for sustaining life and repairing trauma to the body, too much of a good thing can be bad. One study notes that *"heightened inflammatory cytokine levels driven by stress may contribute to depression symptoms by contributing to cell death in brain regions involved in the regulation of mood and emotion"* (Pascoe et al. 2021).

Fortunately, meditation has been shown to lower cortisol (Hopper et al., 2019)

- **Meditation may boost the immune system.** One study involving 30 women found that those who meditated had levels of Immunoglobulin A (IgA, an important protein created by the immune system to find and neutralize pathogens) that were significantly different from those who didn't meditate: "The mean s-IgA titer in the experimental group at 'post-meditation' and '1-hour later' time-points were found to be statistically different from those of the control group" (Torkamani et al, 2018). In other words, mantra meditation may lead to better immunological outcomes.

- **Meditation can change the way you perceive stressors.** This meta-study found important changes in self-compassion, stress response, and other parameters: "Meditation practices are shown to influence many psychological processes that can influence an individual's psychological response and relationship with stressors, including self-compassion, rumination, exposure, metacognition and attention" (Pascoe et al, 2021). Through meditation and mantras, you will shape the way you perceive any health issues you may have. A change in perception and less stress may result in better decision-making and steps in the right direction.

In summary, by meditating on these mantras, you'll hopefully greatly reduce your stress levels, decrease chronic inflammation loads, lessen anger, and even alleviate symptoms of trauma. The many exercises will help you feel grounded, placing you in a state that's more receptive to each mantra.

How to Get the Most Out of This Book

This isn't a work of fiction. It's not a self-help book (although you may find help from reading this book). This is a tool to help you access your inner core and speak to it so that you can make changes in your life that make you a stronger, healthier you. You can jump around from section to section, you can come back to certain mantras, and you can even skip over mantras that don't speak to you.

The point is to leverage this book so that it works for you—maybe you will read the book through in its entirety, or maybe you just prioritize the sections that are most relevant to you. In general, to reap the benefits of the mantras, it's important that you follow some (or all) of the following six steps.

1. **Repeat, repeat, repeat.** When learning anything, it's important to employ a strategy that leverages "spaced repetitions." In other words, it's important to expose yourself to these mantras more than just once or twice. To truly learn something, you've got to repeat reviews over a period of time. For example, you might read a mantra and re-read it the following day, then the next week, then the following week thereafter.

2. **Keep an open mind.** It's important to question your beliefs. Many have built their identities around beliefs that may not be true, or that may be more nuanced than previously realized. For example, you may believe "I'll always be unathletic." I'm asking you to keep an open mind. To be willing to push yourself. To expand or contract your definition of "athleticism", for example. Be open to change.

3. **Do the exercises.** Reading the mantras, and repeating them, can take you far, but the exercises can really help you to make meaningful changes. Most of the exercises are based on powerful meditation techniques I've acquired over the years and can help you find the stillness required to make changes.

4. **If you fall off course, remember you can come back to this book** (if you've only got the eBook, get the physical copy too. Keep it somewhere visible). Always remember that mistakes and poor decisions can arise. Forgive yourself quickly. You're human. Just remember

you can pick this book back up again and start fresh. It may help to keep this book in a physical place to remind you of your commitment to change.

5. **Write it out on a piece of paper.** Writing things down can improve your retention. If there's a mantra that you just want to make stick, getting it down on your own piece of paper can be a great way to do so. Go ahead and grab your favorite pen, or colored pencils, and write down as plainly or creatively the mantras you'd like to adopt.

I hope this book inspires you to take actions that lead to a better you, all while lowering your stress levels and improving your sense of agency. You're capable of change, and I hope you adopt this belief throughout this process. Now, it's time to dig into some mantras!

I Am Capable of Change Right Here, Right Now

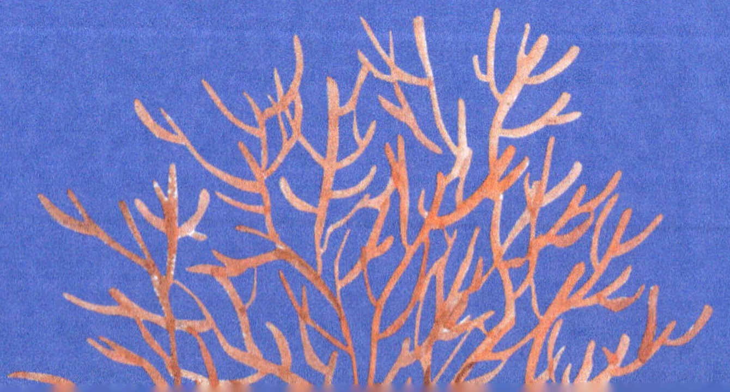

I Am Capable of Change Right Now

Mantras to Inspire Change and Action

"How wonderful it is that nobody need wait a single moment before starting to improve the world"
— Anne Frank

It can be scary walking down this new path of reforming your beliefs—especially if you've struggled with chronic diseases, weight issues or other severe issues. You may feel discouraged, overwhelmed, and hopeless, but you've just got to trust the process. Think of changing your subconscious mind like running a software program on your computer. Software programs take a while to download into the hardwired mind of the computer. Similarly, it's going to take time for your subconscious mind to take what you're telling it seriously.

The installation of this software may fight you at first. Your demons may surface. Little voices in your head may emerge like, "This is pointless" or "I'll never reach ideal health." You've got to silence those voices! You're much stronger than you think. All you need is a bit of activation energy; a few seconds of courage, to prime your subconscious mind.

As we've discussed, your subconscious mind has been programmed from birth. It may take a while for the subconscious mind to accept what you tell it as the truth - but hang in there! It will!

While I acknowledge it'll be hard, it'll be worth it! Imagine living a life where you wake up feeling refreshed and energized every single morning. Imagine days without achy joints. Imagine fitting into old clothes you've outgrown. You've got to keep these end goals in mind to overpower the little voices in your mind that try to put you back on your comfortable (and unhealthy) path.

Promise yourself that you'll start. Right now. Not tomorrow! Not five minutes from now. Not next year.

Not on New Year's Day. Now! You've got nothing to lose and everything to gain! This may not be a perfect time. You may feel terrible and unprepared; your family feast may be this weekend. You may have had pancakes and 10,000 calories this morning. It doesn't matter. You're in exactly the right place and at the right time to receive this message. Forgive yourself for any actions you've taken that may have harmed your health and start anew. Your journey begins now.

There's No Better Time Than Right Now to Be the Healthiest Version of Myself

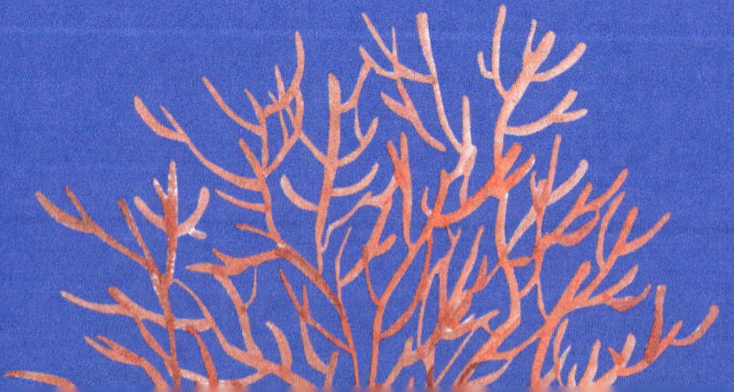

There's No Better Time Than Right Now to Be The Healthiest Version of Myself

This may not seem like a good time to start, but it is. Right now, at this very moment. You can become the healthiest version of yourself. While it may seem counterintuitive, it's vital to create change even if you don't feel you're ready. You may never *feel* ready; this is a mind-over-matter situation. Use your intellect to trust the feelings of ease will come later.

You'll eventually find your groove as your subconscious mind begins to prime you for healing and your choices reflect this change. Even if you're bedridden or are facing a diagnosis with little hope, it may seem like everything is beyond your control. But one thing you can control is your desire to change at this moment. Choose to change now.

Embody this Mantra:

1. Begin drawing your attention to your nose. Feel your breath pass in and out.

2. After a few breaths, doing nothing to change your breathing, close your eyes.

3. Next, imagine a lever in your mind. Shift it to the "on" position. This represents your willingness to start seeing yourself as healthy, and actually being healthy.

4. Feel the change in your body. Do you feel tingles? Warmth? Coolness? Whatever you feel is fine. Pay attention to the passing sensations in your body.

I Surrender My Worries and Believe My Health Is Changing for the Better in This Moment

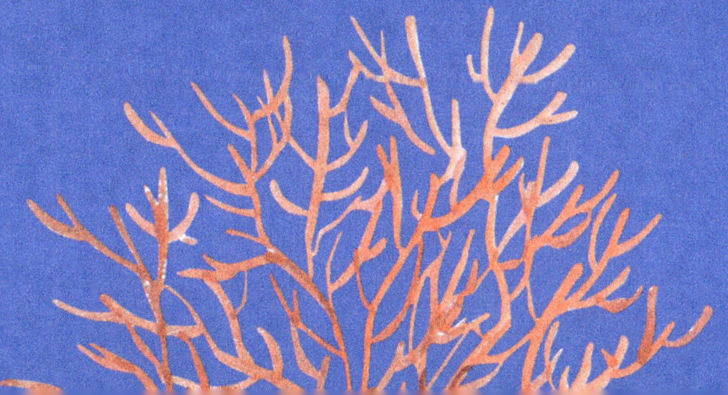

I Surrender My Worries and Believe My Health Is Changing for the Better in This Moment

Now that you've accepted that you're capable of change, this has already begun to chip away at the layers of worry enshrouding your most ideal self. The subconscious mind prefers comfort and security. That's why it'll take some effort from your rational thinking-mind to prod the subconscious mind into a state of growth, necessary for your well-being.

Just by believing in your radical ability to change, you're paving the way for progress. These powerful suggestions are already helping you to create new, tremendously positive habits that can lead the way to creating new neural pathways in the brain.

Rather than stressing about the process, surrender to it. While your conscious mind may not feel your health is changing for the better after accepting this mantra, it is. Belief is a powerful tool, and multiple studies show those who believe they will get better often do. Your enunciation of this mantra is creating shockwaves into your subconscious mind.

Embody this Mantra:

1. Breathe in slowly, filling your abdomen and chest.
2. Exhale your breath, completely deflating the lungs
3. With your lungs deflated, say "My health is improving in this moment"
4. Next, observe the sensations in your body without judging them

My Thoughts and Actions Align to Foster Healing in My Loving Body

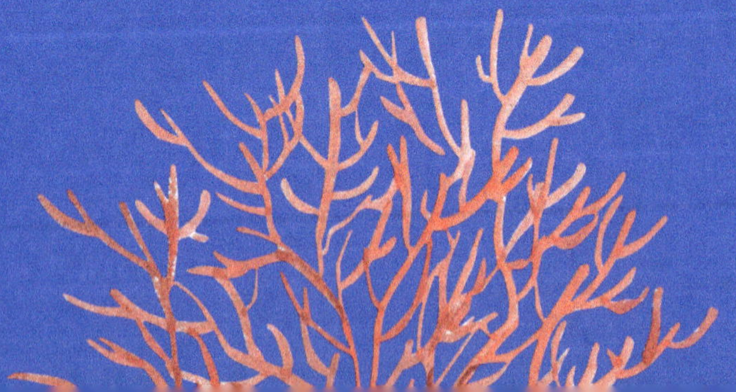

My Thoughts and Actions Align to Foster Healing in My Loving Body

Have you ever wanted to press snooze after your alarm clock goes off? Let's be real, we probably all have at some point! It may seem like you can catch up on a few extra minutes of sleep, but in reality, dozing off an extra few minutes does little to benefit your feeling of restfulness. In a parallel way, now that you've awoken to the powerful benefits of reprogramming your subconscious mind, you can't just lay there—it's time to start your journey!

You've got to promise yourself that you'll start aligning your thoughts with your actions. Suggest to your body that these mantras aren't just mere words, but action plans. These mantras help guide new and improved behavior. They're not just mindless words to enunciate emptily. Taking action can be as little as reading over these mantras regularly, or as big as giving up takeout most nights and investing in a crockpot (who doesn't love crockpot meals?!). The key is to take regular action, no matter how small.

1. Take a deep breath, keeping the eyes open.

2. Observe the breath entering and exit the nose.

3. Raise your right arm upon exhaling, hold, then lower it back to your side as you exhale. Repeat this process on the other side.

4. If you're up for a challenge, head to YouTube and practice yoga. This way, your movements and breaths will become better aligned.

Healing is Easy

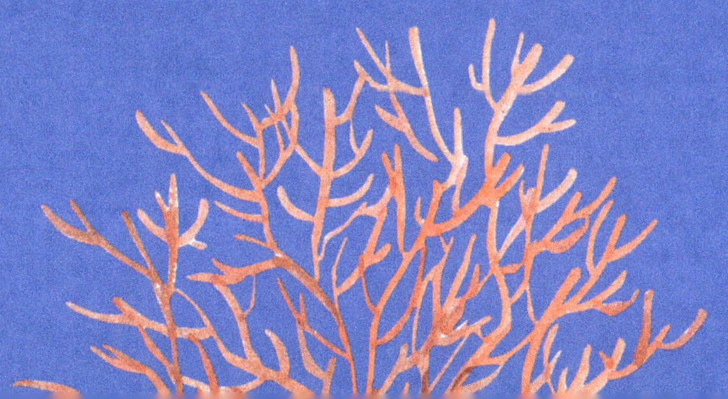

Healing is Easy

"Ease" is the natural state of the body. "Dis-ease" generally emerges when we repeatedly overlook signals from our mind and body. If you've been neglecting to take care of your body for years by eating lots of sugar, trans fats, inflammatory seed oils and drinking soda, your body will scream out to you through skin issues, digestive problems or general malaise. You'll find healing is easy once you learn to listen and respond appropriately to these signals.

When you cut your finger, do you find it difficult to heal it? No, because this healing process is dictated entirely by the subconscious mind. You've got to entrust your subconscious mind as your healing guide. Forget about marketing hype for "new" health products and listen to what nutrients your body is calling out for. Once you take out inflammatory inputs, your body can begin to heal.

Embody this Mantra:

1. Close your eyes in a quiet room.

2. Begin observing the breath, breathing normally.

3. Imagine yourself in a thick Jell-o, unable to move. Feel your arms and legs struggle against the thick substance. Next, imagine the gelatin warming up, becoming liquid, freeing you from stagnation.

4. Focus your mind's eye on swimming with ease. See yourself swimming freely.

My Healing Starts Now

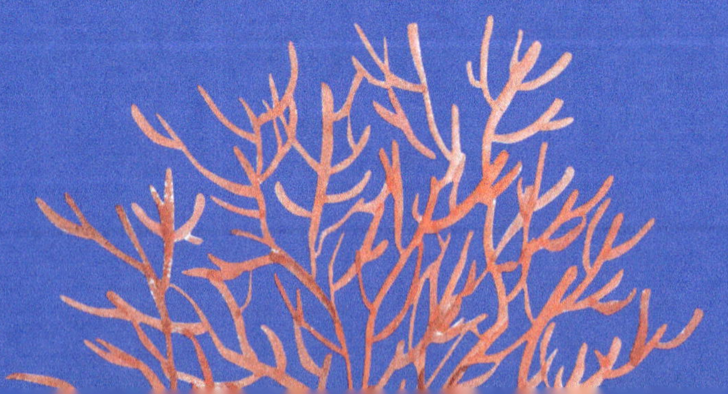

My Healing Starts Now

Continuing the cut finger metaphor, when you cut your finger, it may not seem so, but your body has already begun to heal. Even if crimson blood leaks from the wound, your intelligent body has sent out red and white blood cells to prevent infection. It's started programming for your blood to start clotting near the site of the injury. It's begun sending stem cells to repair the damaged skin. Later, it will be healed as if no injury was ever there.

That's what happens when you accept that healing starts now. Adopting an optimistic outlook is associated with longevity and better disease outcome (Schiavon et al, 2017; Jacobs et al, 2021). The first step is to entrust your body to heal. Healing starts now.

Embody this Mantra:

1. Breathe in slowly, filling your abdomen.
2. As you breathe in, imagine a stoplight with red, yellow and green lights.

3. Envision the green light turning on. Next, imagine the red and yellow lights converting to green and turning on.

4. Continue breathing and see your body being filled with green light.

5. Exhale and say to yourself: "Healing starts now"

Even Though I May Not Feel or Look My Best, I Know I Will

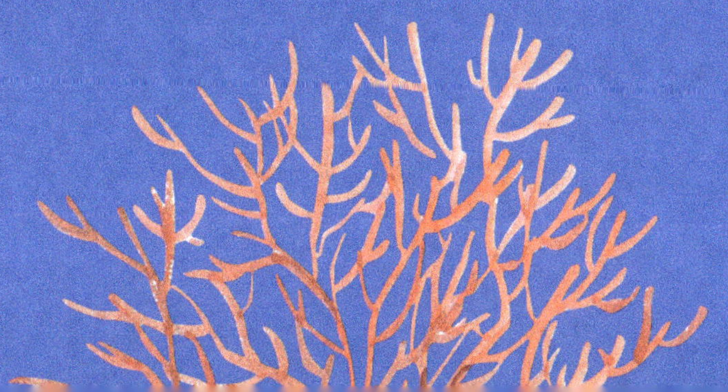

Even Though I May Not Feel or Look My Best, I Know I Will

While there are plenty of benefits of being healthy beyond enhanced physical attractiveness and an increased *feeling* of well-being (for example, increased lifespan, increased healthspan, diminished risk of acquisition of diseases, both chronic and acute, and more), these are two of the most recognized and sought after benefits of exiting a diseased state.

Note that this mantra doesn't read "I feel my best and I look my best" as if it were true in the present. That's because many have mental roadblocks to accepting the ideal image of themselves. We can all be a little self-deprecating; noticing our every flaw. So starting with this baby step, know that your most beautiful, radiant, and energetic self is just around the corner.

Embody this Mantra:

1. Take a deep breath.

2. Affirm to yourself: "Even Though I May Not Feel or Look My Best, I Know I Will"

3. Exhale all self-doubt. Imagine breathing out a toxic gas.

My Journey to My Healthiest Self Has Already Begun

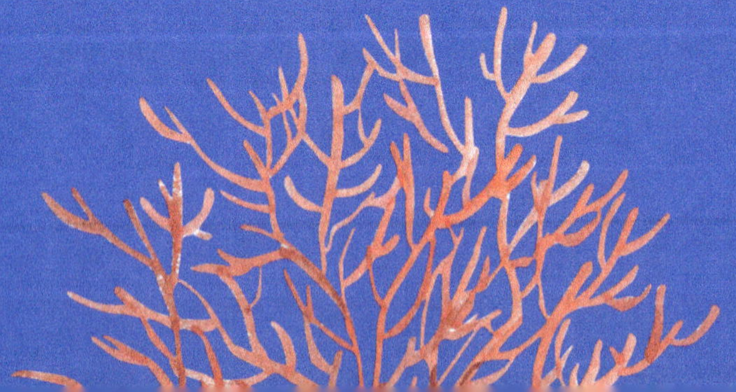

My Journey to My Healthiest Self Has Already Begun

Whether you downloaded this book online or ordered a physical copy, you've already sent messages to your subconscious mind that you value yourself and your health. There are metaphysical benefits that go beyond the content you absorb from this book. Just by deciding to act and picking up this book, you're acknowledging your desire to change and thus your journey to reaching your healthiest state has begun.

You may not have realized the powerful effects of purchasing these books alone - you probably purchase things all the time - but when you think about it, we cast votes with our dollars. Most of us trade our time and energy (the most valuable resources in the world!) for dollars, so by exchanging dollars for products and books that benefit us, we are communicating to our subconscious mind our desire to change for the better and reach our ideal state.

Embody this Mantra:

1. Sit comfortably in a quiet room.
2. Soften your gaze and breathe normally.
3. Envision the startline of a race way in the distance.
4. Look down at your feet and tell yourself: " My healing journey has already begun"
5. Feel gratitude at how far you've gone.

When I Affirm "I Am Healing" I Am Communicating With the Trillions of Cells In My Body To Repair Themselves for the Better

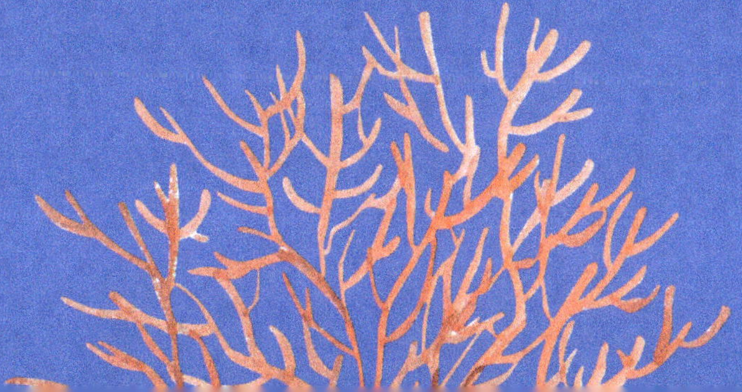

When I Affirm "I Am Healing" I Am Communicating With the Trillions of Cells In My Body To Repair Themselves for the Better

There are metaphysical responses to your thoughts—using mantras has the power to influence minuscule living entities such as your cells and the hormones that live within you. But not only is your inner world influenced by thought alone. In fact, many quantum physicists propose that our thoughts and intentions are able to manipulate the physical world.

This can be affirmed by the many studies that find those who pray face far greater chances of recovering when facing serious health outcomes. One study involving 151 middle-aged patients who underwent cardiac surgery and prayed experienced significantly less depression and less distress than those who did not pray (Ai et al, 1998). This means praying or reciting mantras, either to the self, or to God, has the potential to improve your recovery. That's exciting news!

Most recent science has found that there are 37 trillion human cells on average in the body ([Ando et al, 2020](#)). Why not show them some love and put them at ease? Your cells work harmoniously together; your state of mind, emotions and self-talk have the power to augment their regenerative capabilities.

Embody this Mantra:

1. Begin to take a deep abdominal breath.
2. Exhale fully, until your lungs flatten.
3. Imagine shrinking down the size of a tiny cell.
4. Start up a conversation with your cells, telling them to heal.
5. Continue breathing and feel peace course through your body.

I Love My Body Now. It Sustains Me. It's My Home. It's Healthy And Beautiful

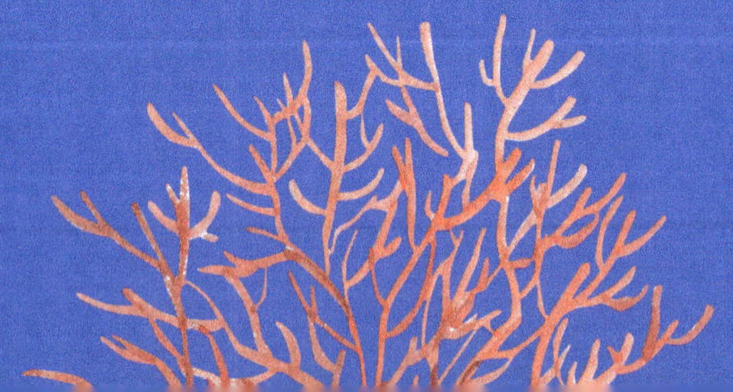

I Love My Body Now. It Sustains Me. It's My Home. It's Healthy And Beautiful

This can be hard to voice for many of you. Many of us have issues with the bodies we live in. We may compare ourselves to people we see in magazines or influencers on Instagram. We might look at our neighbors' glistening grass with envy. Rather than taking action to water our own grass, we may instead satisfy this anxiety (at least in the short run) by adopting a defeatist attitude: 'My grass will never be so green.'

Self-love isn't something that comes easy in an image-based society. With this mantra, your focus should be on accepting your body as is. This means expelling any judgments of the self you may have and opting for an objective view of your body instead. Your body does so many beautiful things! Even if the body seems to be hurting you or has cast disease upon you, really, it's just responding to the inputs you've provided it and is doing its best to sustain you and keep you alive. For that, you should be thankful and show it some love.

1. Take a deep breath in.
2. Hold at the top for three seconds.
3. Release your breath fully.
4. On your next breath in, fill your body with the feeling of love. If you struggle with this, think of someone you love and imagine the sensation overcoming your body.

You Made It!

Thank you so much for making it through this mantras and affirmations book! I hope it inspires you to make positive changes in your life and fills you with a sense of security in your home: your body. I hope you feel less stressed about the ambiguity and the uncertainty you may be facing. I hope you've adopted a new way of approaching any challenges you may be facing along your healing journey. I hope you become the best version of yourself, all while laughing and loving along the way.

If you found this book useful, please leave a quick review (this is extremely important!) and tell a friend. This way others may also begin to adopt a healing mindset through the use of affirmations and mantras, too.

Other books I've written you might also enjoy:

- [Journey On: How to Travel the World - Even If You're Young and Broke](#)

Thanks again for reading. I hope you found, and continue to find, these mantras useful.

About Me

I'm Ryan Scott Shannon, a former fast-paced world traveler turned slow-paced, travel-within type. As of writing this at the end of 2022, I've just finished my master's in work and organizational psychology from the University of Seville (yes, in Spain. Yes, in Spanish). Like just about every other Gen-Zer, I'm trying to escape a corporate career and the 40-hour work week (there's more to life than work and money, right? Where's the time for passions, for rest, for pursuing actualization? For connection?)

While I don't travel as much as I used to, I love teaching people about how to travel cheaply and more authentically via books, ecourses and blog posts. Beyond travel, I'm deeply passionate about psychology after confronting and healing my wounds from my turbulent childhood. I now plan on becoming a licensed professional counselor and plan on writing books that provide people with grounding tools (such as this one).

To see more of my books, click here.

I've also launched Ryan Scott Coffee Table Books which features a collection of children's books, puzzle books and more. Check it out.

Thank You

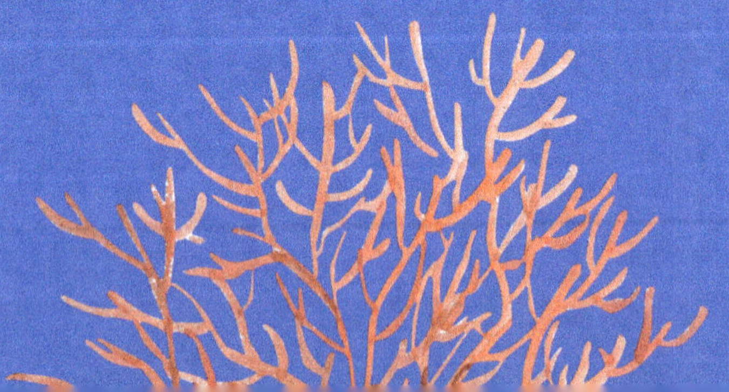

Works Cited

Ai, A. L., et al. "The Role of Private Prayer in Psychological Recovery among Midlife and Aged Patients Following Cardiac Surgery." *The Gerontologist*, vol. 38, no. 5, 1 Oct. 1998, pp. 591–601, 10.1093/geront/38.5.591. Accessed 8 Feb. 2020.

Ando, Yoshinari, et al. "An Era of Single-Cell Genomics Consortia." *Experimental & Molecular Medicine*, vol. 52, no. 9, Sept. 2020, pp. 1409–1418, 10.1038/s12276-020-0409-x. Accessed 2 Mar. 2022.

Barbuzano, Javier. "Understanding How the Intestine Replaces and Repairs Itself." *Harvard Gazette*, 14 July 2017, news.harvard.edu/gazette/story/2017/07/understanding-how-the-intestine-replaces-and-repairs-itself/.

"Consumer Expenditures in 2020 : BLS Reports: U.S. Bureau of Labor Statistics." *Www.bls.gov*,

www.bls.gov/opub/reports/consumer-expenditures/2
020/home.htm.

Dempersmier, Jon, and Hei Sook Sul. "Shades of Brown: A
Model for Thermogenic Fat." *Frontiers in
Endocrinology*, vol. 6, 8 May 2015,
10.3389/fendo.2015.00071. Accessed 6 Dec. 2019.

Fox, Kieran C.R., et al. "Functional Neuroanatomy of
Meditation: A Review and Meta-Analysis of 78
Functional Neuroimaging Investigations."
Neuroscience & Biobehavioral Reviews, vol. 65,
June 2016, pp. 208–228,
10.1016/j.neubiorev.2016.03.021.

Furness, J. B., et al. "Nutrient Tasting and Signaling
Mechanisms in the Gut. II. The Intestine as a
Sensory Organ: Neural, Endocrine, and Immune
Responses." *The American Journal of Physiology*,
vol. 277, no. 5, 1 Nov. 1999, pp. G922-928,

pubmed.ncbi.nlm.nih.gov/10564096/,

10.1152/ajpgi.1999.277.5.G922.

Hopper, Susan I., et al. "Effectiveness of Diaphragmatic Breathing for Reducing Physiological and Psychological Stress in Adults." *JBI Database of Systematic Reviews and Implementation Reports*, vol. 17, no. 9, Sept. 2019, pp. 1855–1876, journals.lww.com/jbisrir/fulltext/2019/09000/effecti veness_of_diaphragmatic_breathing_for.6.aspx, 10.11124/jbisrir-2017-003848.

Hülsheger, Ute R., and Hugo J.E.M. Alberts. "Assessing Facets of Mindfulness in the Context of Work: The Mindfulness@Work Scale as a Work‑Specific, Multidimensional Measure of Mindfulness." *Applied Psychology*, 2 Dec. 2020, 10.1111/apps.12297.

Hyland, Patrick K., et al. "Mindfulness at Work: A New Approach to Improving Individual and Organizational Performance." *Industrial and*

Organizational Psychology, vol. 8, no. 4, 15 July 2015, pp. 576–602, www.cambridge.org/core/journals/industrial-and-org anizational-psychology/article/mindfulness-at-work-a-new-approach-to-improving-individual-and-organi zational-performance/881148F1CFDB6C1E2FEECF 4962389599, 10.1017/iop.2015.41.

Jacobs, Jeremy M, et al. "Optimism and Longevity beyond Age 85." *The Journals of Gerontology: Series A*, vol. 76, no. 10, 20 Feb. 2021, pp. 1806–1813, 10.1093/gerona/glab051. Accessed 28 Dec. 2022.

Lin, Lifeng. "Bias Caused by Sampling Error in Meta-Analysis with Small Sample Sizes." *PLOS ONE*, vol. 13, no. 9, 13 Sept. 2018, p. e0204056, 10.1371/journal.pone.0204056.

Malaktaris, Anne, et al. "Higher Frequency of Mantram Repetition Practice Is Associated with Enhanced Clinical Benefits among United States Veterans with

Posttraumatic Stress Disorder." *European Journal of Psychotraumatology*, vol. 13, no. 1, 10 June 2022, 10.1080/20008198.2022.2078564. Accessed 5 Sept. 2022.

Oman, Doug, et al. "Mantram Repetition as a Portable Mindfulness Practice: Applications during the COVID-19 Pandemic." *Mindfulness*, 16 Nov. 2020, 10.1007/s12671-020-01545-w.

Pascoe, Michaela C., et al. "Psychobiological Mechanisms Underlying the Mood Benefits of Meditation: A Narrative Review." *Comprehensive Psychoneuroendocrinology*, vol. 6, May 2021, p. 100037, 10.1016/j.cpnec.2021.100037. Accessed 24 Mar. 2021.

Schiavon, Cecilia C., et al. "Optimism and Hope in Chronic Disease: A Systematic Review." *Frontiers in Psychology*, vol. 7, 4 Jan. 2017,

www.ncbi.nlm.nih.gov/pmc/articles/PMC5209342/,
10.3389/fpsyg.2016.02022.

"Topic: Pharmaceutical Industry in the U.S." *Www.statista.com*, Statista, 2008, www.statista.com/topics/1719/pharmaceutical-industry/.

Torkamani, Fatemeh, et al. "Effects of Single-Session Group Mantra-Meditation on Salivary Immunoglobulin a and Affective State: A Psychoneuroimmunology Viewpoint." *EXPLORE*, vol. 14, no. 2, Mar. 2018, pp. 114–121, 10.1016/j.explore.2017.10.010. Accessed 10 Feb. 2020.

Whitehead, Ross D., et al. "Attractive Skin Coloration: Harnessing Sexual Selection to Improve Diet and Health." *Evolutionary Psychology: An International Journal of Evolutionary Approaches to Psychology and Behavior*, vol. 10, no. 5, 20 Dec. 2012, pp.

842–854, pubmed.ncbi.nlm.nih.gov/23253790/. Accessed 28 Dec. 2022.